I0830713

$12.99 US

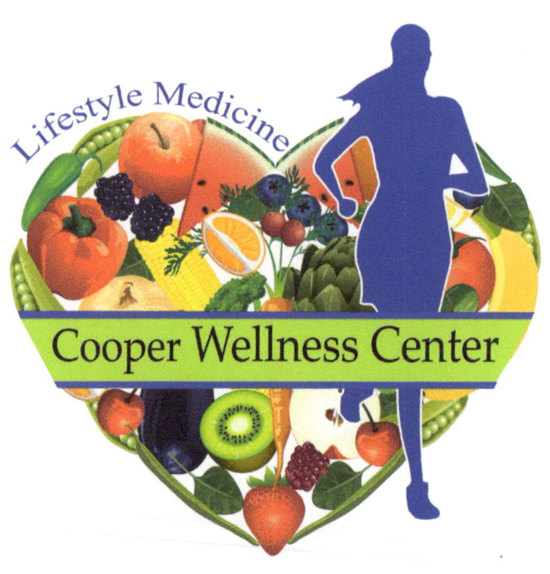

Get Healthy with Dr. Cooper™
3604 N. McColl Road
McAllen, TX 78501
www.Gethealthywithdrcooper.com
Copyright ©2018 by Dona Cooper-Dockery, M.D.

All Biblical quotations, unless otherwise noted, are taken from The Holy Bible, New King James Version (NKJV).

Copy edited by: LaKesha Brooks
Cover design and interior design by: Debra Marcketti

ISBN 978-1-7232-5278-5

Printed in the U.S.A.

CONTENTS

Introduction

Though science is progressing in its discoveries, our health as a nation is not improving. Obesity has become an epidemic in the USA. At least 2 in 3 adults are either overweight or obese (NIH, 2017). Childhood obesity has tripled in the U.S. since the 1970s. One in three American school-aged children and teens is either overweight or obese (American Heart Association). Diseases that once older adults suffer are now the fare of younger generations. Diabetes, high blood pressure, cardiovascular disease and cancers are rampant, taking many to an early grave.

What is the cause of this health crisis? While chronic diseases like hypertension, cardiovascular diseases, and diabetes have a genetic component, (you have a higher risk of them if a first or second degree relative has had them), they are not wholly caused by genetics. The scientific literature is filled with overwhelming evidence that unhealthy lifestyle practices, especially poor food choices, are the cornerstone of these chronic diseases that plague our nation. Our lifestyle plays a greater role in the development and prevention of diseases than genetics. As it is said, "Genetics load the gun, lifestyle pulls the trigger". As a result, in the majority of cases, when it comes to chronic diseases, HEALTH IS A CHOICE; it is not predestined.

What is the solution? The solution is certainly not another pill—else our health problems would have been long resolved! The solution is adopting a healthy lifestyle, since poor lifestyle is the culprit. You CAN today choose to revolutionize your health, become free from diseases, by changing your lifestyle! Many others have done it successfully and you can too!

The objective of this work manual is to share with you in a succinct way that optimal lifestyle that will help you get well, stay well, enjoy vibrant energy, and all your God-given potential.

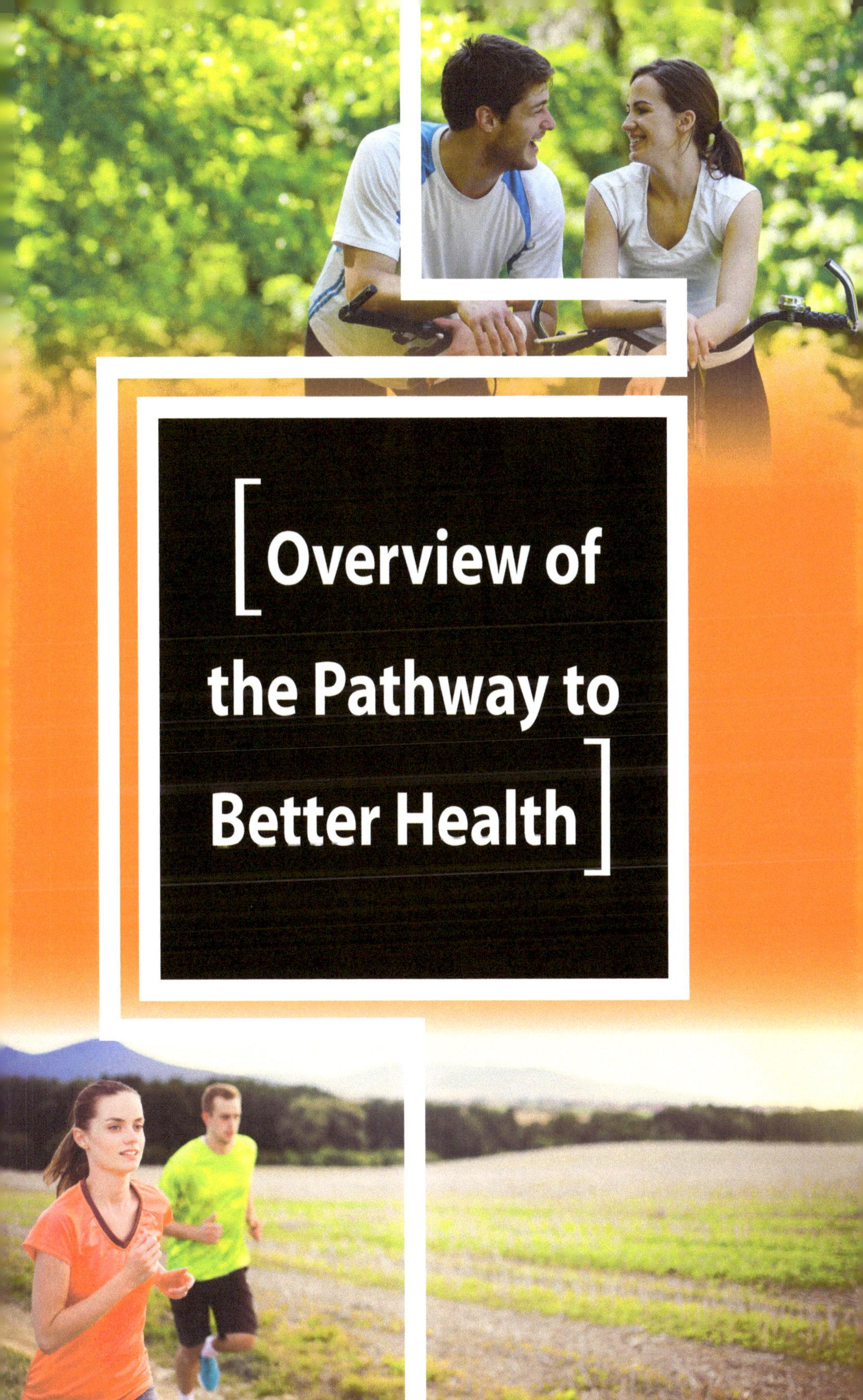

[Overview of the Pathway to Better Health]

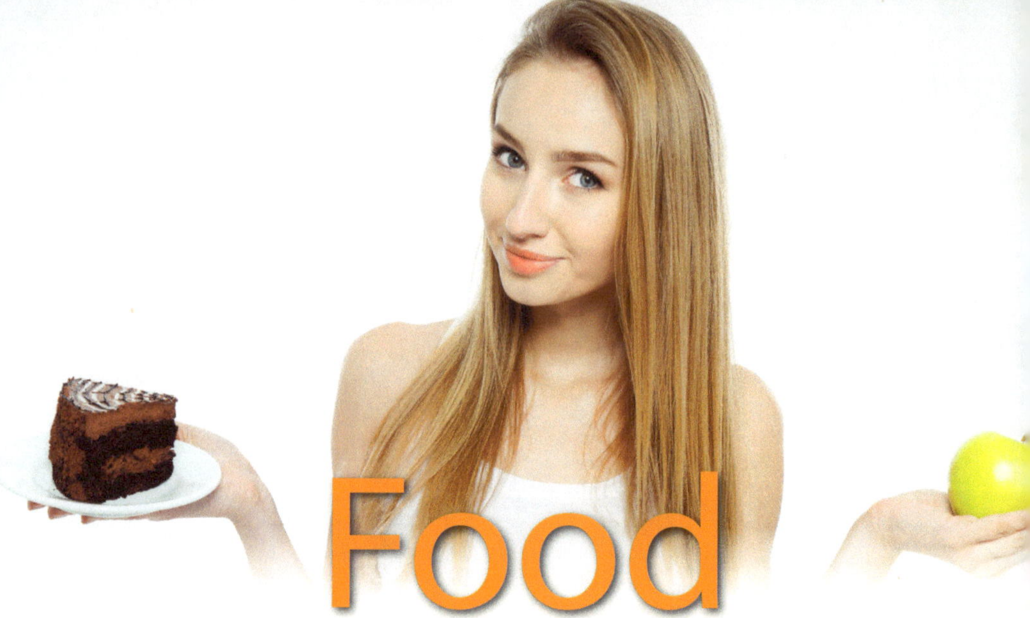

Food

Food is the number one risk factor for diseases. This was established over two thousand years ago by Hippocrates. He said "Let food be thy medicine and thy medicine be thy food". The Global Burden of Diseases Study, the most comprehensive analysis on the causes of death, published in 2012, also confirmed that **our diet is our biggest killer!**

Here is a list of foods that can be hazardous to our health:

1) Processed meats (bacon, hot dog, ham, salami, sausage, deli meats), other meats, and fish

2) Dairy and eggs

3) Animal fat in general and most oils

4) Stimulants, such as alcohol, coffee, caffeinated drinks, chocolate

5) Sodas and other sugary drinks

6) Snacks (candy bars, chips, and other fried foods)

7) Refined foods (like sugar, white flour, white pasta, white bread, white rice)

8) Too much salt (One with hypertension should not take more than ½ teaspoon of salt a day. It is best to use Himalayan salt or pure sea salt rather than table salt)

Health Foods

1) Fruits. According to the Global Burden of Disease Study aforementioned, not eating enough fruit is the number one dietary problem that can shorten one's life

2) Vegetables (leafy greens, non starchy vegetables like broccoli, and root vegetables and beets and carrots)

3) Whole grains and their derived whole-grain flour (brown rice, barley, rolled oats, quinoa, rye, spelt, millet, whole grain bread, whole grain pasta, whole grain flour).

4) Legumes (black beans, lentils, chickpeas, etc) and tubers (sweet potatoes, yuca)

5) Nuts and seeds

6) Plenty of water

We will discuss in more detail the benefits of each of these food groups in the upcoming sections.

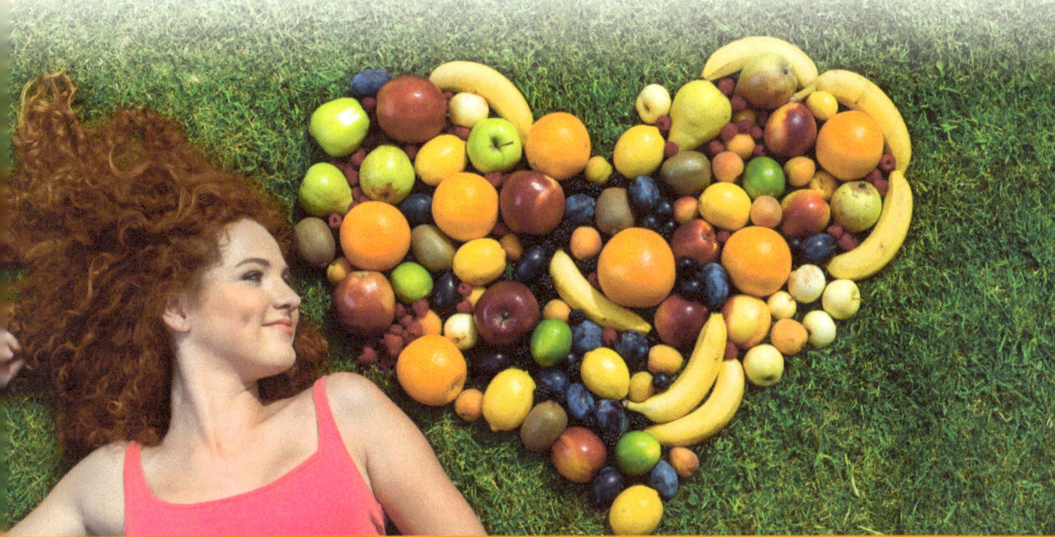

Healthy Pantry

GRAINS:
barley
brown rice
bulgur wheat
couscous
millet
multigrain cereal
oats (old-fashioned, rolled)
rye
spelt
quinoa
tortillas
whole-grain bread
whole-grain flours
whole-grain pastas
wild rice

FLOURS:
cornmeal
whole wheat
wheat bran
oat
chickpea
brown rice
rye
barley
spelt
soy
vital gluten wheat germ

NUTS & SEEDS:
almond
cashew
chia seeds
coconut
pecans
pumpkin seeds
sesame seeds
sunflower seeds
walnuts
flaxseeds
whole flaxseed

LEGUMES:
black beans
black-eyed peas
garbanzo beans (chickpeas)
navy beans
kidney beans
pinto beans
lima beans
lentils
red beans
soybeans
split peas
peanuts

NUT BUTTERS:
almond butter
cashew butter
peanut butter
tahini

DRIED HERBS & SPICES:

allspice
sage
basil
rosemary
cayenne pepper
Italian seasoning
celery seeds
cumin
curry powder
onion powder
garlic powder
ground cinnamon
McKay's chicken-style seasoning
Mrs. Dash herbal seasoning
nutritional yeast flakes
turmeric
oregano
coriander
sea salt
cinnamon

DRIED FRUITS:

cranberry
dates
figs
prunes
raisins

FRUITS & VEGETABLES:

fresh fruits and vegetables of all varieties and colors

CANNED ITEMS:

beans
light coconut olives
tomato paste pimentos
vegetable broth

EQUIPMENT:

blender
food processor
waffle iron

Meats

PROCESSED MEATS

The consumption of processed meat is directly linked to an increased risk of diseases, such as cancer and coronary heart disease. Processed meats are meats preserved using the following methods: curing, salting, smoking, or adding chemicals, such as sodium nitrite. Some examples of processed meats include bacon, ham, salami, hot dogs, corned beef, bologna, sausage, beef jerky, etc. Research now shows that the consumption of meats preserved with nitrites or nitrous compounds increases the risk for developing cancer, especially cancer of the stomach and colon. Other harmful chemicals, such as polycyclic aromatic hydrocarbons, are formed during the smoking of meat. These chemicals are also produced during barbecuing, grilling, and roasting. These harmful compounds are transferred from wood, coal, or hot surfaces into the air before accumulating on the surface of the meat products and are also cancer-causing agents. Salting of meat, an old practice, is also dangerous as a diet high in sodium increases the risk of hypertension, which in turn increases the risk of heart disease and death.

WHAT'S WRONG WITH OTHER MEATS?

According to the U.S. Department of Agriculture, the average American will consume 222.2 lbs. of red meat and poultry this year (2018) compared to 129 lbs. in 2012. That is a lot of meat, especially in the light of all the research studies that encourage us to refrain from animal foods. For years, many studies have proven that eating meat once or more days a week significantly increases the rates of diabetes. The more frequently meat is eaten, the higher the risk of the disease. Researchers at Harvard Medical School conducted a study that included 120,000 candidates that proved that a diet high in red meat can shorten life expectancy by increasing one's risk of death from cancer and heart-related problems. Avoiding both processed and unprocessed meat will decrease your risk of dying early from some cancers and cardiovascular diseases. Is it just the red meat and processed meat? The Adventist-2 study, which looked at 89,000 people, showed that the more plant-based a diet is (that is, the lesser meat, fish, or other animal products it contains), the lower the rate of diabetes. In this study, there was a 78% lower prevalence of diabetes among those eating strictly plant-based! In the Taiwan study published in 2014, Taiwanese who ate very healthy (no processed foods, no sugar) but ate a small portion of meat just once a week had greater rates of diabetes than those who ate less meat, while the vegan ones in the study (who ate no animal food) had no diabetes at all. It is in the best interest of one who wants to overcome diabetes to let go of animal products altogether (including chicken, fish and dairy) A plant-based diet has been shown to be more effective in the management and reversal of diabetes than the diet prescribed by the American Diabetes Association.

Eating any type of animal products increases the workload on the kidneys within hours of consumption, while plant protein does not cause any issues. One may still obtain enough protein after removing animal products from their diet. We do not need a large amount of protein in our diet to be in good health. Adults require no more than 0.8 or 0.9 grams of protein per healthy kilogram of body weight per day. Another easy way to calculate protein need is to take one's ideal weight in pounds, multiply it by four, and then divide it by ten. For instance, someone whose ideal weight is 100 pounds will require up to 40 grams of protein a day. Even when you remove all animal products from your diet, there is nothing to fear; you will find enough protein in fruits, vegetables, nuts, grains, and seeds. We are more likely to suffer from protein excess than protein deficiency. There are many adverse effects associated with long-term high protein diets, especially when the protein is from animal sources like meat, milk, cheese or eggs. Some of the disorders from excess protein intake include disorders of bone and calcium balance, impaired kidney function, chronic kidney disease, increased cancer risk, diseases of the liver, and worsening of coronary artery disease. Plant protein is associated with less hyperfiltration and protein leakage, and therefore prevents or slows down the deterioration of our kidneys.

Furthermore, animal products have no fiber, which is very important for a healthy body. We will discuss the benefit of fiber in the next segment. While they have no fiber, they are rich in cholesterol which can jeopardize your health, especially your heart. Plant foods do not contain cholesterol; only animal products do. We do not need to consume cholesterol from our foods because our bodies naturally produce their own cholesterol. Eating animal products will cause an abnormal increase in cholesterol level, in high blood pressure, and in your risk for stroke. Animal foods are also void of antioxidants and phytochemicals that help us fight free radicals, as well as prevent and reverse diseases. As if this was not enough, there is also the big concern of steroid hormones in animal products, both the hormones that are naturally occurring in the animal as well as the synthetic hormones that are injected in them for business purposes, to increase milk production for instance. Because of this, the consumption of animal products has the potential of increasing the hormone IGF-1 in the body, which in turn may increase your risk for cancer and the progression of cancer in one already diagnosed. Hormones in meat can also decrease a woman's fertility, while milk and its products may lower sperm count in men, increase the risk for prostate cancer, trigger type 1 diabetes in children, as well as early puberty (which equates greater cancer risk).

The risks associated with animal products are too great, especially considering that they are not essential to our health. We can get all the nutrients our bodies require from plant sources. The oldest recorded research study on the impact of animal products on our health also supports the fact that animal products are not optimal for health. The findings of this study are recorded in the first chapter of the book of Daniel (one of the books of the Bible). In Daniel chapter 1, four young men ate a completely plant-based diet and drunk water, while the rest of their peers (the control group) followed a diet that contained animal products and wine. After 10 days, the group that ate only plants (fruits, vegetables, etc.) and water was found to have an intellectual quota TEN TIMES higher than the control group. In other words, they were ten times wiser and smarter. The plant-based diet did not only positively impact their mind but also their physique. It is reported that just after ten days on a whole food plant-based diet, their countenance was fairer and healthier. Try it yourself! Just ten days feasting on plant foods while staying away from health hazardous products (animal and processed foods) can get you on a journey to feeling and *looking* your best!

Protein Content in Whole Grains	
Types of Whole Grains	**(1 Cup Cooked) Grams of Protein**
rye	25
sorghum	22
spelt	11
amaranth	9
farro	8
quinoa	8
wheat	7
whole wheat pasta	7
wild rice	7
buckwheat	6
bulgur	6
millet	6
oats	6
brown rice	6
corn kernel	6
barley	4
whole wheat bread	4
white bread	4

Protein Content in Beans & Legumes	
Types of Beans & Legumes	**(1 Cup Cooked) Grams of Protein**
soy nuts (soya beans)	68
lentils	18
edamame	17
red kidney beans	16
adzuki beans (red beans)	15
black beans	15
chickpeas (garbanzo beans)	15
pinto beans	15
Anasazi beans	14
fava beans	13
lima beans	12
pigeon beans	11
black-eyed peas	5
butter beans	5
peanuts	5

The usual recommended daily amount of protein is 0.8mg/kg; the average person with a weight of 75 kg will have a need of 60 mg daily.

Fats

Fat is an essential component of a healthy and balanced diet. Fats help keep the body warm, provide energy, participate in cell growth, aid in the absorption of fat-soluble vitamins (A, D, E, and K), in the production of important hormones, and are essential for blood clotting and muscle movement. The problem with fats is the type and the amount of fats one consumes. The healthy fats are derived from plants while the bad fats are usually from animal sources or are man-made (trans fats).

SATURATED FATS

Saturated fats are primarily from meat, milk, cheese and eggs. Coconut and palm oils are plant sources of saturated fats. Saturated fats can increase total cholesterol level and LDL (the bad cholesterol), which in turn increases the risk for heart disease and type 2 diabetes. A diet high in animal products may increase your cholesterol in the long run. Some studies recommend the consumption of lean meats not more than twice weekly while others suggest total abstinence from all animal products for optimal health (as we have seen already).

TRANS FATS

Trans fats, often referred to as the worst fats, are produced when a vegetable oil is hydrogenated to become semisolid or solid fat. (They are man-made). They are found in butter, shortening and products containing them (cookies and other baked goods). In food labels, such as some peanut butter brands, they are listed as "partially hydrogenated oil" or "hydrogenated oil". They too can increase LDL (the bad cholesterol), while suppressing HDL (the good cholesterol). They create inflammation, increase the risk of heart disease and stroke, contribute to insulin resistance, which in turn increases the risk of diabetes. According to the Harvard Health Publishing, they are harmful even in very small amount—every 2% of calories from trans fat taken daily increases the risk of heart disease by 23%!

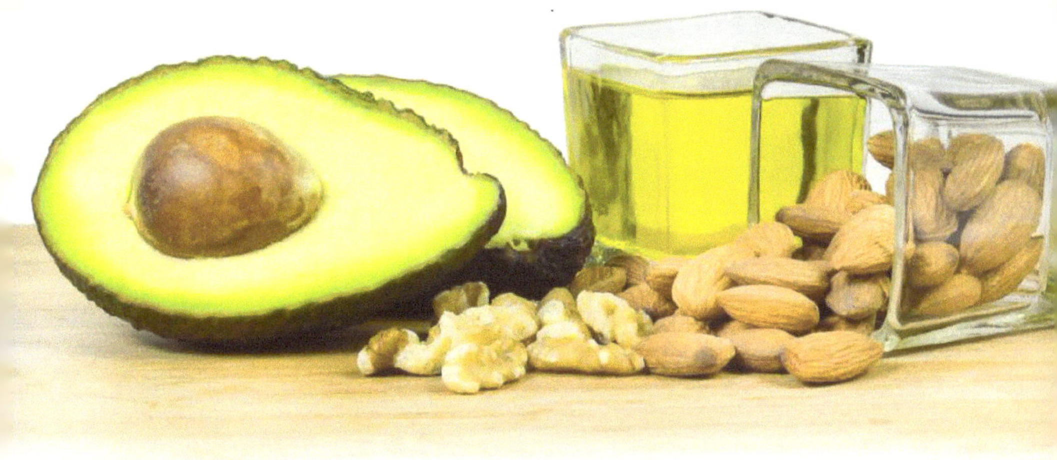

Healthy Fats

Healthy fats come from plants, such as nuts, seeds, avocados, and olives. They are cholesterol free, help lower the bad cholesterol (LDL) and increase the good cholesterol (HDL). Nuts and seeds are very nutritious. They are natural hunger-busters, not only because of their fat content, but also because of their healthy protein and fiber content. As a result, when consumed in moderate amounts, they may also help with weight control. Not much is needed to get their benefits: just a handful of nuts five times a week may help protect the heart—it is about five ounces a week. One ounce or 2 tablespoons of flaxseeds will provide 7.5 grams of fiber, while an ounce of almond nut will provide 3.5 grams of fiber, which promotes regularity and glucose control.

Omega-3 fatty acid are one type of healthy fats that is especially beneficial to the heart, by decreasing the risk for coronary artery disease. Some excellent sources of omega-3 are flax seeds, chia seeds, walnuts, and sunflower seeds.

TIPS ON USING HEALTHY FATS

1) Avoid animal products (meat, dairy, and cheese) as they are high in saturated fat and calories but low in nutrients and fiber

2) Avoid partially hydrogenated or hydrogenated oils (read your labels to know if the product you are buying contains them)

3) Eliminate butter, margarine or lard. You may use vegetable oil but in small quantities as too much vegetable oil means excess calories that may lead to weight gain. For instance, just one tablespoon of olive oil provides 120 calories. It is possible to prepare tasty foods without the use of oil.

4) Consume a handful of nuts five days a week and/or two to three tablespoons of ground flax, chia, or pumpkins seeds daily

5) One gets the most benefits out of flax seeds if they are eaten ground. However, it is best not to buy your flax already ground as flax meal oxidizes quickly on the shelf. Buy your seeds whole and grind them in a dry blender (or grinder) before eating. You may also freeze your homemade and freshly ground flax meal to preserve it for future use.

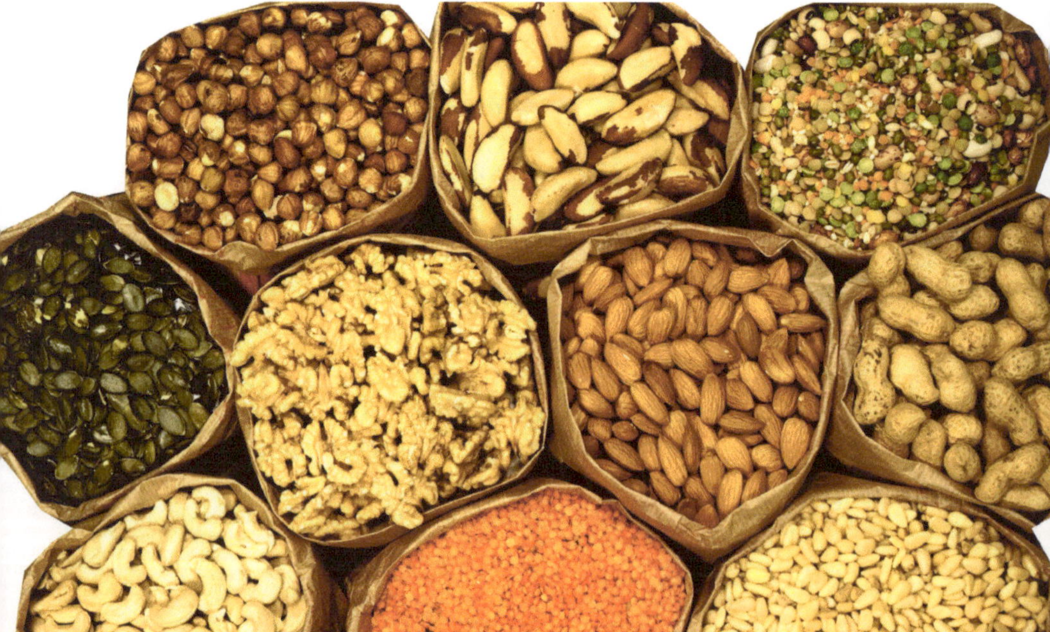

Whole Grains

Whole grains are becoming more popular as more are realizing their health benefits. They help reduce the risk of coronary artery disease, may help to prevent, improve or reverse diabetes. They also provide various types of nutrients that are important for proper body function. Yet, there is still much misinformation on grains, even as far as some "experts" calling them toxic foods. The issue with grains is the type or the quality. Are the grains you consume whole grains (unprocessed) or are they refined (processed)? This is an important question to ask yourself when you think of purchasing grains.

A grain is composed of three main parts:

- bran, which is the fibrous shell and contains the most nutrients
- endosperm, also known as the kernel, makes up the bulk of the grain and contains a small amount of vitamins and minerals
- germ, which is the smallest part of the grain but contains lots of nutrients and healthy fats.

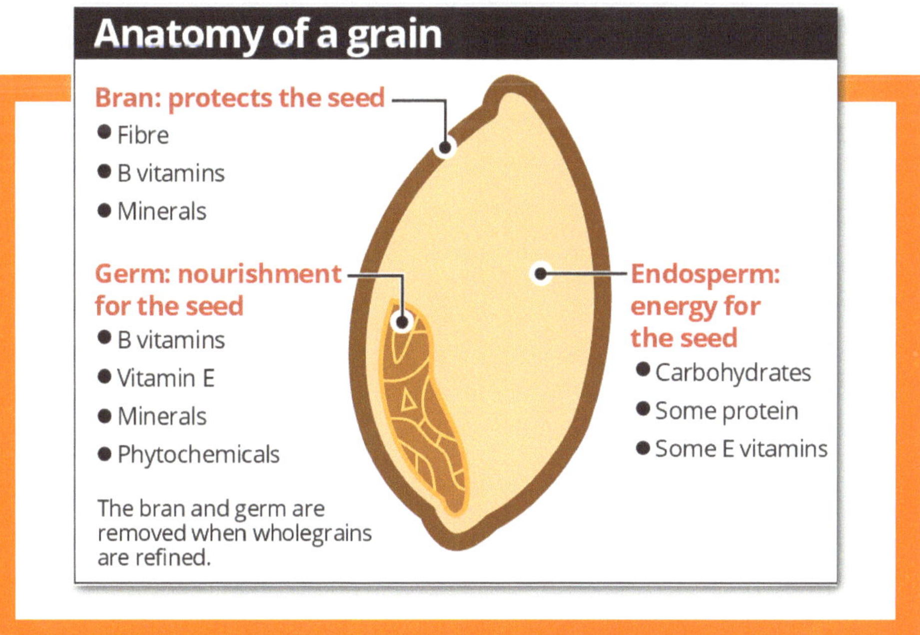

When a grain is processed, the bran and the germ are removed, leaving behind the endosperm, which is mainly carbohydrates with few vital nutrients. Processed grains are left mostly with the carbohydrate portion while losing some of its fiber, vitamins, minerals and phytonutrients. The milling process removes iron, B complex vitamins, and fiber. The lack of fiber in processed grains contributes to blood sugar spikes in diabetics, leads to constipation, causes the food to be less filling and thereby leads to eating more food and more calories, which may ultimately contribute to weight gain.

With enriched grains, about twenty essential nutrients are removed from the whole grain and five of them are added back. If someone steals twenty dollars from you and gave you back five dollars, they certainly did not "enrich" you. Enriched grains are still inferior to whole grains in terms of the quality of nutrients they provide as well as the health benefits that these grains offer. Some grains are fortified, which means nutrients that don't occur naturally in the food are added in. On the other hand, WHOLE grains provide essential nutrients, such as vitamin E, thiamine, iron, and magnesium, as well as fiber and antioxidants. To promote optimal health, it would be well to consume primarily whole grains. Some examples of whole grain products are brown rice, quinoa, barley, rye, millet, wheat berries, bulgur, and corn.

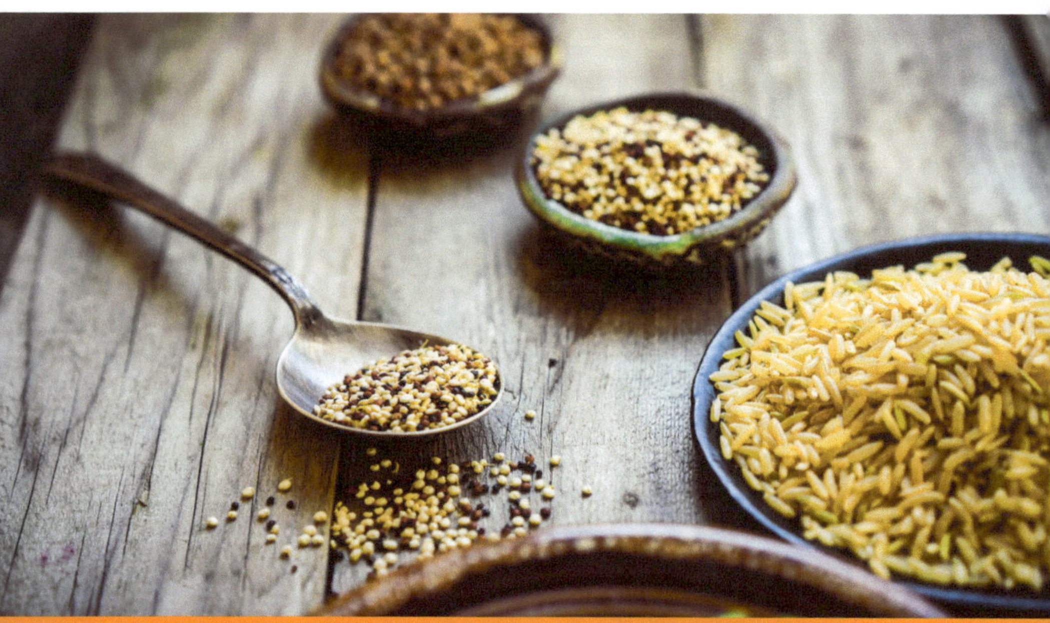

Benefits of Fiber

The higher fiber content in whole grains assists in slowing glucose absorption. This will decrease the glucose spike seen in diabetics and therefore will lead to better glucose control. It may even lead to a reversal of diabetes. For example, there is a greater risk of diabetes with consumption of white rice versus the use of brown rice.

Fiber also has more bulk. It remains longer in the stomach. This keeps you feeling fuller longer, which then decreases the need to snack between meals. Consuming foods high in fiber, such as whole grains, is a great way to lose weight and maintain a healthier weight. Fiber is also great to lower LDL cholesterol. It gives bulk to the stool, which is important for regular bowel movements. Regular bowel movements reduce the risk of constipation and the formation of diverticulosis, which results from high pressure within the large intestines producing bulging pouches in the lining of the bowel. As a result, whole grains lower total cholesterol, lower LDL (low-density lipoprotein), triglycerides, insulin levels, decrease the risk of clots, heart attacks, and other cardiovascular diseases. (Remember that we shared earlier that animal products have ZERO fiber; which means that you miss out on all these protective benefits of fiber when you consume animal foods). Whole grains, by providing higher fiber can also help decrease the risk of colon cancer.

Read your label

A "whole grain" stamp on food items does not always mean healthy grain. The item may contain both whole grains and processed grains. Therefore, learn to read food labels carefully and purchase those items that are 100 percent whole grains.

How to increase whole grain consumption

Where possible, use whole grain rather than whole grain products. For example, choose wheat berries over whole wheat crackers. Serve brown or wild rice at mealtime. Add brown rice or barley to your soups. Add variety to your diet by discovering other whole grains such as rye, quinoa, or millet. Choose whole-grain products (100% whole grain breads, pasta, etc).

Legumes

Legumes, such as beans, peas, lentils, constitute an inexpensive and excellent source of protein, complex carbohydrates, minerals (such as iron and zinc), vitamins, fiber, and antioxidants. They are an ideal substitute for meat.

Unlike animal products, there are free of saturated fats, which helps protect against coronary artery disease and lower blood pressure. Just half a cup of legumes may give a third of daily fiber requirements. In most cases, 1 cup of cooked legumes provides 33 percent protein for females and 28 percent for males. Because of this, they help prevent and cure constipation, prevent diverticulosis and hemorrhoids, as well as achieve and maintain a healthy weight and lower blood cholesterol level. They also have a low glycemic index that will not cause a rapid surge in blood sugar levels. They can be added to salads or soups. They can be sautéed, spiced, and served over brown rice. They can be made into dips like hummus.

With the high fiber content of legumes, they are not completely digested and some people may experience some intestinal discomfort and gas production (flatulence) because of this.

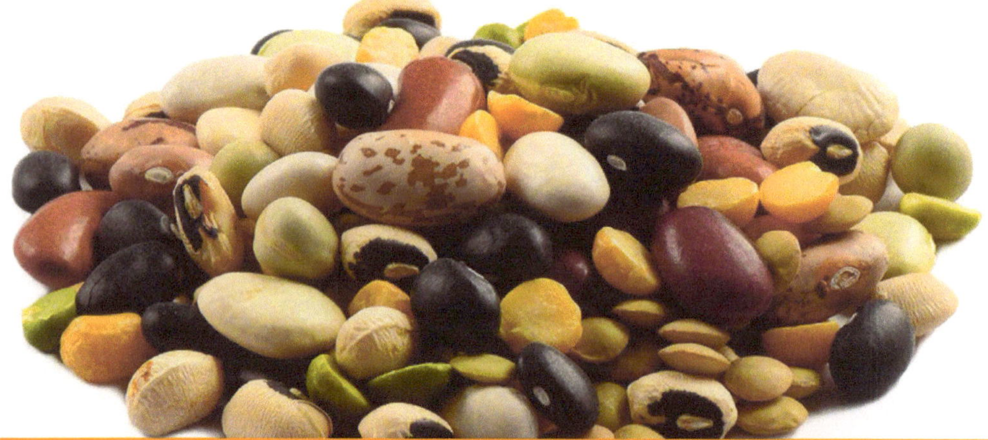

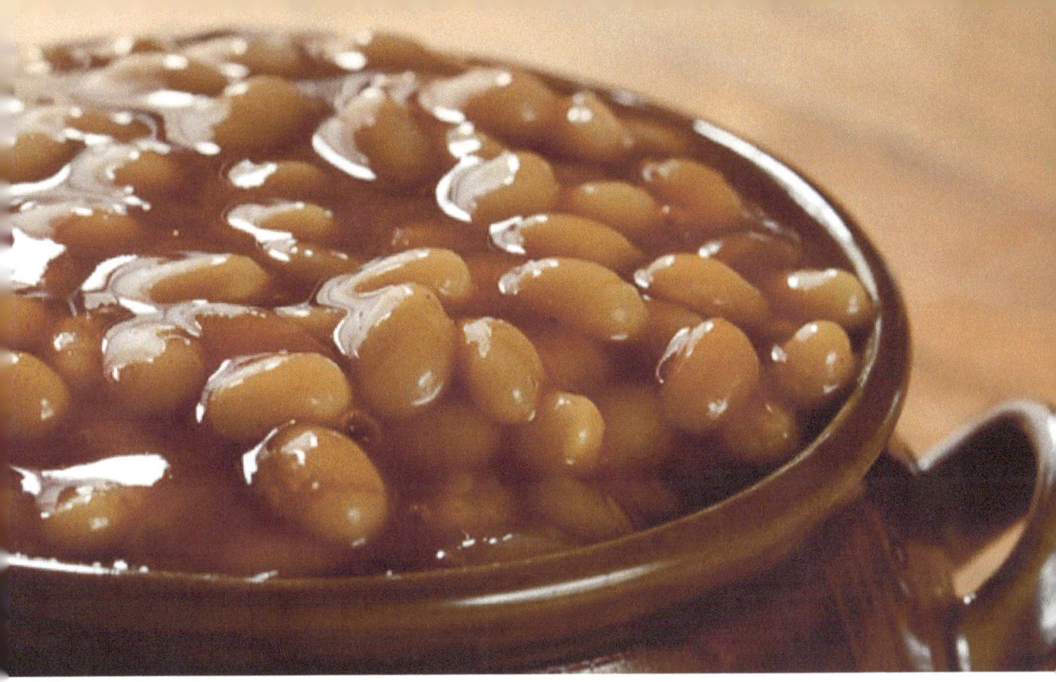

TO REDUCE THE INTESTINAL DISCOMFORT, HERE ARE SOME TIPS:

1) Soak packaged raw legumes overnight, or at least for a few hours before cooking. Then before cooking them, discard the water in which they were soaked and rinse them off and cook with fresh water

2) Sprouting your legumes is another option. In addition to improving digestion, sprouting may also increase the nutritional content of your legumes

3) When using canned beans, you should pour off the water and rinse before cooking.

4) Consume a handful of nuts five days a week and/or two to three tablespoons of ground flax, chia, or pumpkins seeds daily

5) If you have not been consuming legumes, then start by introducing a small amount to your meal— two to three tablespoons. This will help your digestive system become used to processing this new food with high fiber. As the flatulence decreases, you can slowly increase the amount of legumes in your diet

Fruits & Vegetables

Fruits and vegetables were an integral part of the original diet given to Adam and Eve that contributed to their long life span.

Vegetables—whether green leafy vegetables, cruciferous and other vegetables—ought to be a focus in our diet. A minimum of five servings of these nutrient-dense foods is recommended daily. Vegetables, especially green leafy vegetables, can help prevent and reverse diabetes. Cruciferous vegetables like kale, collard greens, broccoli, cauliflower, cabbage, Brussel sprouts, are excellent in fighting cancer. Other greens and non-starchy vegetables, like spinach, romaine lettuce, eggplant, onions, garlic have almost nonexistent effects on blood glucose and are packed with fiber and phytochemicals. They are also very low in calories; therefore, they are excellent for weight loss or maintaining a healthy weight.

Fruits are low in fat, sodium, and calories, while they are high in fiber, folic acid, potassium and vitamin C. We have explained in detail the benefits of fiber in the section on whole grains—from regularity in bowel movement, weight control, to cancer prevention. Fruits, being high in fiber offer all these benefits. Adequate intake of potassium as provided in fruits helps maintain healthy blood pressure. Vitamin C is important for the growth and repair of all body tissues, helps heal cuts and wounds, and keeps teeth and gums healthy. Folic acid helps form red blood cells and is crucial for women of childbearing age to prevent neural defects in the developing fetus. Citrus fruits (oranges, limes, grapefruits, berries, papaya, and cantaloupe) are good sources of folic acid and vitamin C. Fruits, such as berries, cantaloupes, pears, kiwis, tomatoes, and plums, are great for diabetics. A minimum of four servings of fruits is recommended daily.

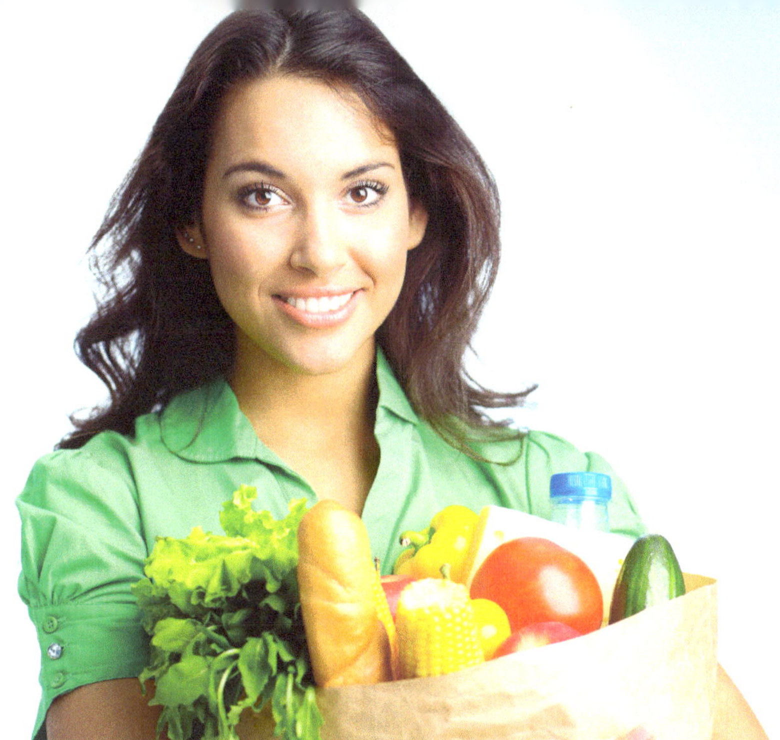

Tips on preparation and consumption

Eat a variety of fruits and vegetables of different colors to benefit from their unique vitamins, minerals, and phytonutrients. Fill at least half of your plate with fruits or vegetables, to obtain a minimum of nine to twelve servings a day of fruits and vegetables. An easy way to achieve this is having fruits or vegetables at each meal and integrating them in your recipes.

For maximum benefit, it is best to consume your vegetables raw (in salads) or slightly steamed. Overcooking the vegetables will lead to loss of essential nutrients, such as vitamins and minerals. Fruits should be consumed whole. When the juice is extracted, most of the fiber will be lost. Commercially prepared juices are high in calories with less antioxidants and nutrients. If you wish to liquefy your fruits, then smoothies are better than juice extraction. With the smoothie, the fiber is also consumed.

The consumption of fruits and vegetables instead of foods such as rice and potatoes will lead to better blood sugar control and will prevent or reverse type 2 diabetes.

Glycemic Index and Load Table

Food Type	GI	GL
glucose	100	10
white potato	85	26
watermelon	72	4
white rice	72	16
white bread	70	10
cantaloupe	65	4
sweet potato	61	17
pineapple	59	7
wild rice	57	16
honey	55	10
maple syrup	54	10
kiwi	53	6
mango	51	8
ripe banana	51	13
brown rice	50	16
whole wheat bread	49	9
grapes	46	8
peach	42	5
white pasta	41	26
strawberry/blueberry	40	1
apple	38	6
pear	38	4
whole wheat pasta	38	17
chickpeas / kidney	28	8
cashew nuts	25	3
cherries	22	3
agave	19	2
cauliflower	15	2
eggplant	15	2

Glycemic Index and Load Table Cont.

Food Type	GI	GL
lettuce, spinach	15	1
soybeans	18	1
tomato, zucchini	15	2
broccoli, mushroom	10	4
cabbage	10	2
kale	2	3

Diabetic patients should choose foods with very low glycemic index in order to improve their health or reverse their disease.

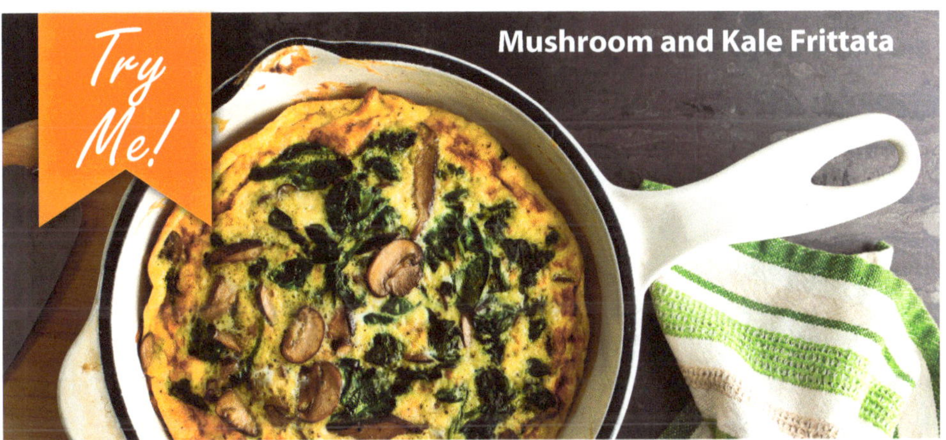

INGREDIENTS:

1 small onion, chopped
2 cups mushrooms
2 cups Tofu Scramble
(See recipe on page 36)
4 cups coarsely chopped kale leaves
2 cloves garlic, mashed & minced
¼ tsp salt
1 cup rolled oats
1 cup soy milk
½ cup whole-wheat flour
½ tsp baking powder
2 tbsp olive oil

PREPARATION:

Blend oats; add in wheat flour, baking powder, baking soda and salt. In a separate bowl mix milk and oil. Then combine both and set aside. Spray large oven proof skillet with nonstick cooking spray; heat over medium heat. Add onion and mushrooms; cook and stir 6-8 minutes or until onion is light golden. Add kale and garlic; cook 3-5 minutes or until kale is wilted. Evenly spread mixture to cover bottom of skillet. Pour Tofu Scramble over Kale mixture. Cover and cook 6-7 minutes or until almost set. Then mix milk, oats, flour and baking powder. Pour mixture over sautéed vegetable tofu, slightly mix. Preheat broiler. Uncover skillet; broil 2-3 minutes or until golden brown and set. Let stand 5 minutes before cutting into 6 wedges.

Exercise

While poor diet is the greatest contributing risk factor to diseases and mortality in the U.S., followed by smoking, physical exercise is still a vital part in a healthy lifestyle plan. Physical inactivity ranks #5 in terms of risk factors for death and #6 among risk factors for disability in the U.S.

Regular physical exercise is not only useful in weight management, but it is also good for health and longevity. Cancer mortality is decreased to less than 50% with vigorous exercise 30 minutes daily. Exercise decreases the risk of diabetes, high blood pressure, heart disease, high cholesterol, depression, and anxiety. It improves the overall quality of life and mood, builds stronger bones, improves immunity, energy, and endurance.

As of 2017 only 21.7% of adults aged 18 and over met the Physical Activity Guidelines for both aerobic and muscle-strengthening activity; which means that 78.3% of the population is not as active as they should. A wise writer once penned these words, "**More people die for want of exercise than from overwork;** very many more **rust out** than wear out" (Christian Temperance and Bible Hygiene, p 101.2). Let us not be among those that rust out! Let's get moving!

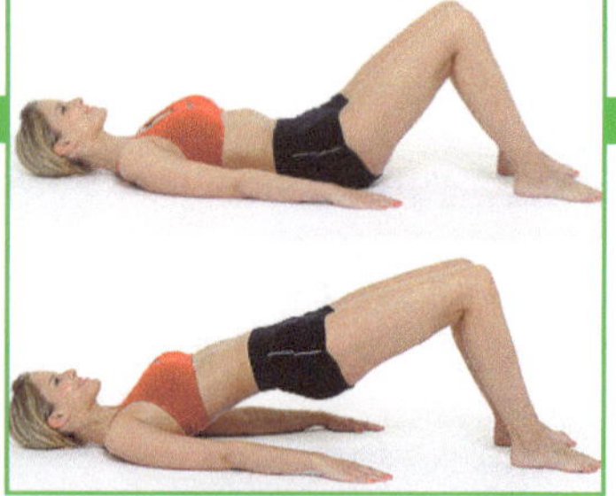

Lie flat on the floor on your back with your hands by your sides and knees bent. Your feet should be shoulder width apart. This is the starting position.

Push primarily with your heels, lift your hips off the floor while keeping your back straight. Once at the top, hold position for a second.

Slowly go back down to the starting position, repeat.

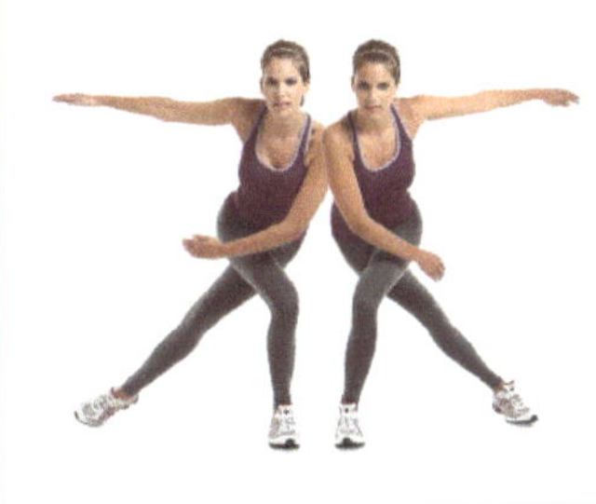

Stand on one leg. Hop from side to side alternating legs as if you were jumping over a tree branch.

Pump your arms side to side reaching above shoulder no higher than head (opposite hand to the standing leg), Knees are slightly bent and body is low. Repeat for 10-20 Reps

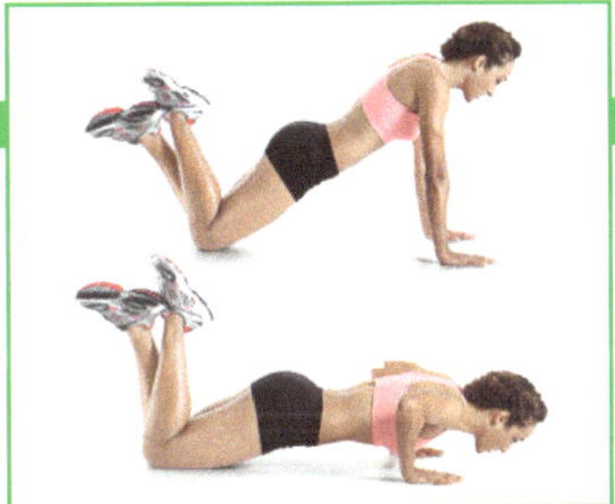

Start in modified push-up position, knees on floor. Keeping abs tight, bend elbows and lower chest toward floor. Press back up to start and extend right arm at shoulder level. Continue alternating arms with each rep.

The recommendation is a minimum of 30 minutes of moderate exercise for six days a week. A rule of thumb to understand moderate exercise is exercise that causes you to break a sweat or exercise during which you cannot sing but can still have a conversation. For a more technical grasp of moderate exercise, one can aim at achieving at least 75 percent of their maximum heart rate. To find this out, just subtract your age from 220; the number remaining is the maximum heart rate. Now the goal is to achieve 75 percent of that number. Let's say that you are twenty years old. Your maximum heart rate would be 200, but the desired heart rate to achieve would be 75 percent of 200, which would be 150. An adequate exercise program should include exercises aimed at improving cardiorespiratory fitness, as well as muscular strength, flexibility, and balance.

TIPS ON MOVING MORE:

1) Pick the goal you hope to achieve, whether weight loss, muscle tone, more energy, better sleep, etc.

2) Choose an activity you may enjoy, whether walking, biking, swimming, etc.

3) Start slow. Begin three to four times a week for ten to fifteen minutes at a time, then increase at least to the minimal requirement of 30 minutes 6 days a week. For weight loss, one hour six days a week is recommended

The best time to exercise is the time that you will be able to commit to in the long run. Exercising in the morning may help prevent its cancellation from the common excuse of being "too busy" or "too tired" during the rest of the day. If you have some chronic illnesses that cause you to be concerned about starting an exercise regimen, then discuss your plans with your health care provider and ask for medical guidance and/ or clearance. Exercise is medicine! Use it!

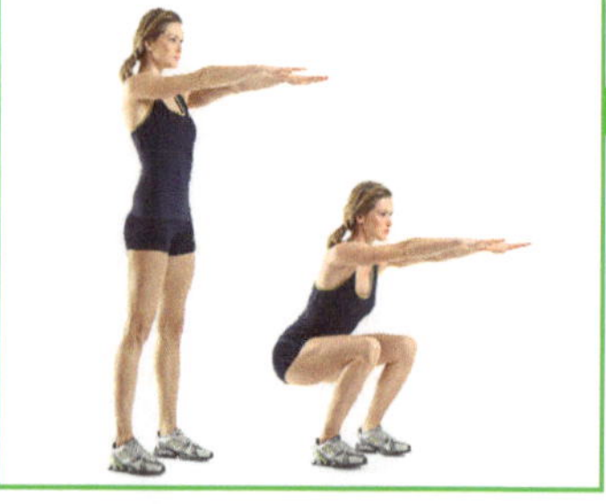

Stand in a shoulder width stance with toes pointed straight ahead. Keeping an upright trunk/torso.

Bending hips back and bending knees will initiate the squat. Lower as far as body can be controlled form, goal is to be at or lower than knee level. Extend the hips, knees, and ankles to return to standing position.

The 12-Week Program

1) Whole food plant-based diet (fruits, vegetables, grains, legumes, nuts and seeds)

2) Two main meals: breakfast as the largest meal and a moderate size lunch. If a third meal is taken, it should be light and small, at about 5 or 6 in the evening, several hours before bedtime to ensure proper digestion before you go to sleep. Sleeping on a full stomach robs your body of the rest it needs and may contribute to weight gain in the long run

3) Eat your fruits and vegetables at the beginning of your meal and make them the centerpiece of your table for weight control and to keep chronic diseases at bay

4) Limit the intake of vegetable oils, sugar, salt, and nut butter (calorically dense)

5) Eliminate processed foods, sodas, coffee, and alcohol

6) Drink plenty of water—half of your body weight in ounces. (For instance, if you weigh 160 lbs., you need half of that number in ounces, which would be 80 ounces of water a day. 1 cup of water has 8 ounces. To get your 80 ounces of water a day, you would need 10 cups a day). Stay away from coffee (damaging to your nervous system), soda, concentrated fruit juices, and other sugary drinks

7) At least 30 minutes of exercise six days a week

8) Spend to to fifteen minutes per day in the sun to boost your vitamin D level (for a stronger immune system and overall good health)

9) Get seven to eight hours of sleep per night. Seek to go to bed preferably no later than 10 PM

10) Spend twenty to thirty minutes daily in bible reading. It will help with stress management, will improve mental and emotional outlook, as well as provide continual inspiration to continue on your health journey

IDEAS WHEN GOING OUT:

a) Select salads with low-fat dressings and without the meats, or request lemon juice as dressing

b) Order a vegetable soup. This is a great way to fill up without packing on the calories

c) Order a bean burrito or pizza using vegetable toppings without the cheese

d) Order a tofu dish at an Asian restaurant or a pasta with marinara sauce at an Italian restaurant

e) Take your friends and family to a vegan or vegetarian restaurant. These restaurants are popping up everywhere now as more people are become more health-conscious!

MORE TIPS FOR SUCCESS:

1) Be mentally ready to start this new healthy lifestyle. Assess your health risks to help you understand your need for a change. Until you see your need for change, you will not be mentally ready for it and will likely not go all into it

2) Then determine your goals (Is it weight loss? Is it blood sugar under 100?)

3) Remove things from your sight that may tempt you to relapse (processed foods, meats, cheeses, etc). Clean up your fridge and kitchen cabinets.

4) List all the fruits and vegetables, whole grains, nuts, and seeds that you enjoy eating. Then learn how to consume these foods in a healthier manner, using less fat, sugar, and salt. For breakfast: Fresh fruits, cooked oats or other whole grains (millet, buckwheat, brown rice) with nondairy milk, granola, or whole-grain bread with nut butter or leftover beans made into a spread. For lunch a fresh salad (fifty percent of your meal), slightly steamed greens or other vegetables, some whole grains and/ or legumes. (You may follow the recipes provided at the end)

5) Make a meal plan and stock up with healthy foods that you enjoy. (When you have gone through my proposed fourteen-day meal plan, you will be equipped to take more control and design your own meal plans)

6) Replace bad habits with good ones. According to the experts, your habits can rewire your brain. When you repeat a task for a long time, your brain maps pathways to cause you to perform that task without thinking about it. The good news is that you can rewire your brain by replacing unhealthy habits with healthy habits. So keep doing what is right (like eating a fruit instead of ice cream or exercising instead of playing video games) and very soon the right habit will become second nature! You can actually bring about change in your brain by introducing a good habit perpetually for as few as seven days. The first place to begin your change process is in your eating habits

7) Take care of your thought life! Research has shown that every thought we process, whether positive or negative, has a physiological response in our bodies. Negative emotions, such as the feeling of anger, hate, or lack of forgiveness, will increase the risk of diseases like hypertension, heart disease, stroke, and even death. In contrast, positive thoughts, such as happiness and hope, are essential for the development of healthy behaviors and thus a happier and longer life

Words of encouragement

Change can be difficult but not impossible. Meditation, prayer, and seeking divine intervention may help to further empower you to make a healthy lifestyle change that will last for a lifetime. You will discover that changing to a healthier lifestyle can be quite exciting and enjoyable with all the new foods and alternatives one gets to try!

There is hope for you beyond diabetes, hypertension, obesity and heart disease! You are not destined to be on medications the rest of your life. Believe it and commit to following a healthier lifestyle one day at a time. The benefits that will follow, both physically and mentally will be beyond what you had hoped for!

How Healthy Are You?

Instructions—For each health indicator, check the box in the column that best describes you. Write the score for that column in the score column on the right.

Health Indicators	Column A 0	Column B 5	Column C 10	Score
Disease—Do you have high blood pressure?	Yes, uncontrolled	Yes, controlled	No	
Disease—Do you have diabetes?	Yes, uncontrolled	Yes, controlled	No	
Disease—Do you have heart disease?	Yes, uncontrolled	Yes, controlled	No	
Body weight—What is your body mass index? (BMI chart on page 35)	BMI 30+	BMI 25–29.9	BMI <25	
Blood pressure—What is your blood pressure?	140/90+	120/80–139/89	<120/80	
Physical activity—Do you engage in at least 30 minutes daily of moderate or vigorous exercise?	No regular physical exercise	2–3 days per week	5–7 days per week	
Fruits and vegetables—How many servings daily do you consume? (1 serving = 1 medium fruit, 1/2 cup cooked vegetables, 1 cup raw vegetables)	0–3	4–5	6–9	
Whole grain—How many servings per day do you consume? (1 serving = 1 slice whole wheat bread, 2/3 cup brown rice, oatmeal, quinoa, or dry cereal)	<1/day	1–2 servings/day	3+ servings/day	

Continued ▶

Health Indicators	Column A 0	Column B 5	Column C 10	Score
Legumes—How many servings of legumes do you have per day? (1 serving = 1/2 cup cooked beans, peas, or lentils)	<1 servings per day	1–2 servings per day	3 or more servings per day	
Nuts and seeds—How many servings do you have per week? (1 serving = 1 ounce nuts or seeds, 2 tablespoons of nut butter)	0–2 servings per week	2–4 servings per week	5 or more servings per week	
Red and processed meats—How many servings of meat do you have per day? (egg, beef, ham, sausage, salami; (1 serving = 3 ounces)	>3 servings per day	1–2 servings per day	<1 serving per day	
Snack foods—How many times per week do you consume candy bars, chips, fries, and sodas?	>7 times per week	2–6 times per week	<1 per week	
Water—How many cups of water do you drink daily?	<5 cups per day	6–7 cups per day	8 or more cups per day	
Breakfast—Do you have breakfast regularly?	Seldom	Sometimes	Daily	
Sleep—What is the average amount of you sleep per day?	5 hours per day	<7 hours per day	7–9 hours per day	
Sugar—What is your blood sugar level, if known?	126+	100–125	<100	
Blood cholesterol—What is your LDL cholesterol level, if known?	160+	130–159	<130	
Smoking status—Indicate your present status.	Current smoker	Ex-smoker	Nonsmoker	

Continued ▸

Health Indicators	Column A 0	Column B 5	Column C 10	Score
Social relationships—Indicate your current status.	Have no social or family support / rarely connect	Some family and social support / connect occasionally	Strong family and social support / frequently connect	
Happiness—How happy are you?	Not happy, often sad or depressed	Somewhat happy / seldom sad	Very happy and satisfied with life	
Time outdoors—How much time do you spend outdoors?	<10 min.	10–30 min. per day	30 or more min. per day	
Hope and the future—What is your outlook on the future?	Pessimistic	Somewhat optimistic	Very optimistic	
Spiritual connection / meditation—Indicate your current status.	No spiritual or religious belief. I do not meditate.	I am learning about spiritual values / meditate often.	I have faith and engage regularly with people of the same faith / I meditate regularly.	

Total lifestyle score _____________

0–60 very high risk	65–100 moderate risk	105–150 average risk	155–200 good	205–300 excellent

NOTES:

____

____

____

____

____

Body Mass Index Chart

Instructions—Use this chart to determine your BMI, and use that number to answer the questions on the previous pages.

	Weight in pounds																
	Normal						Overweight					Obese					
4'10"	91	96	100	105	110	115	119	124	129	134	138	143	148	153	158	162	167
4'11'	94	99	104	109	114	119	124	128	133	138	143	148	153	158	163	168	173
5'	97	102	107	112	118	123	128	133	138	143	148	153	158	163	168	174	179
5'1"	100	106	111	116	122	127	132	137	143	148	153	158	164	169	174	180	185
5'2"	104	109	115	120	126	131	136	142	147	153	158	164	169	175	180	186	191
5'3"	107	113	118	124	130	135	141	146	152	158	163	169	175	180	186	191	197
5'4"	110	116	122	128	134	140	145	151	157	163	169	174	180	186	192	197	204
5'5"	114	120	126	132	138	144	150	156	162	168	174	180	186	192	198	204	210
5'6"	118	124	130	136	142	148	155	161	167	173	179	186	192	198	204	210	216
5'7"	121	127	134	140	146	153	159	166	172	178	185	191	198	204	211	217	223
5'8"	125	131	138	144	151	158	164	171	177	184	190	197	203	210	216	223	230
5'9"	128	135	142	149	155	162	169	176	182	189	196	203	209	216	223	230	236
5'10"	132	139	146	153	160	167	174	181	188	195	202	209	216	222	229	236	243
5'11"	136	143	150	157	165	172	179	186	193	200	208	215	222	229	236	243	250
6'	140	147	154	162	169	177	184	191	199	206	213	221	228	235	242	250	258
6'1"	144	151	159	166	174	182	189	197	204	212	219	227	235	242	250	257	265
6'2"	148	155	163	171	179	186	194	202	210	218	225	233	241	249	256	264	272
6'3"	152	160	168	176	184	192	200	208	216	224	232	240	248	256	264	272	279
6'4"	156	164	172	180	189	197	205	213	221	230	238	246	254	263	271	279	287
BMI	19	20	21	22	23	24	25	26	27	28	29	30	31	32	33	34	35

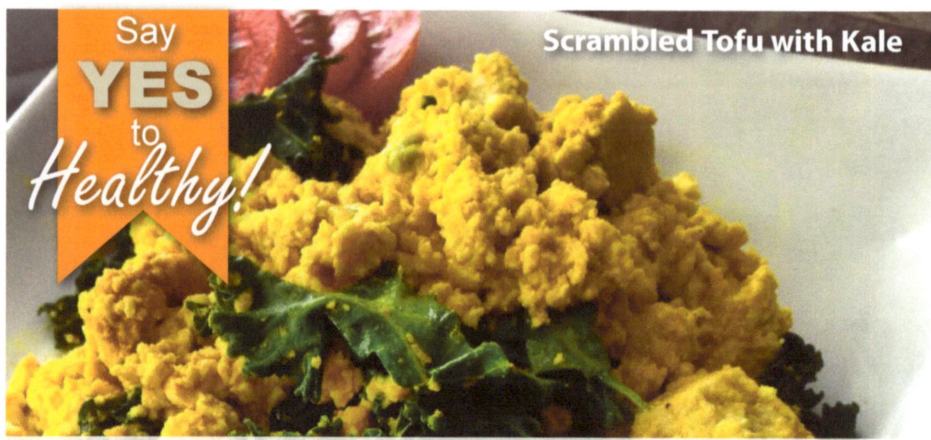

Scrambled Tofu with Kale

INGREDIENTS:
1 (16-oz) package water-packed, extra-firm organic tofu
½ cup chopped onion
¼ cup bell peppers
½ cup tomatoes
4 cups kale, coarsely chopped
2 tsp savory seasoning
½ tsp turmeric powder
½ tsp salt
½ tsp onion powder
½ tsp garlic powder
½ tsp thyme
2 tsp Mrs. Dash Seasoning
2 tsp vegetable oil

PREPARATION:
Remove the tofu from its package, rinse, drain, and set aside. In large skillet/ sauce pan, saute the onion, peppers, and other spices for 5 minutes in hot oil. Scramble tofu in skillet and add remaining ingredients, except kale. Allow to cook for 7 minutes on medium heat. Add kale. Stir occasionally. Cover until kale is wilted, about another 3-5 minutes. Serve with whole-wheat bread, baked potatoes or over brown rice.

Avocado Toast

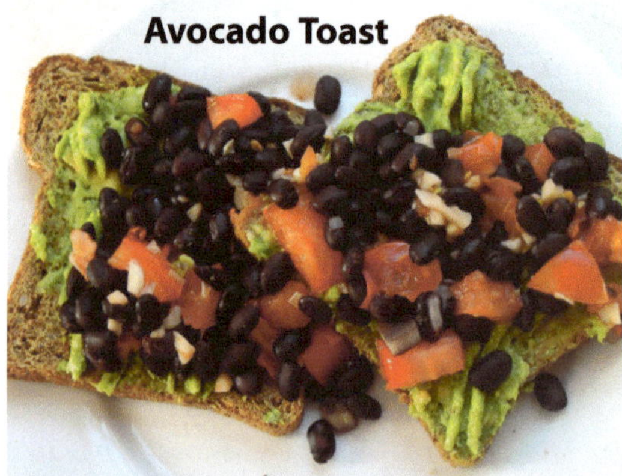

INGREDIENTS:
4 thick slices of multi-grain bread
1 ripe avocado
¼ cup lime juice + pinch of salt
1 large sliced tomato
½ cup black beans (warmed)
½ small red onion, chopped

PREPARATION:
Mash avocado with a fork until smooth, sprinkle salt, add onion and lime juice. Toast bread, then spread the avocado and add sliced tomato and spoonful of black beans for added protein.

NOTES:

SOME ADDITIONAL REFERENCES USED:
- https://www.health.harvard.edu/staying-healthy/the-truth-about-fats-bad-and-good
- https://www.ncbi.nlm.nih.gov/pubmed/23245604
- https://nutritionfacts.org/2016/02/02/the-number-one-global-diet-risk/
- https://www.bloomberg.com/news/articles/2018-01-02/have-a-meaty-new-year-americans-will-eat-record-amount-in-2018
- http://www.ncbi.nlm.nih.gov/pubmed/24523914
- https://nutritionfacts.org/audio/how-much-is-enough-protein/
- https://www.ncbi.nlm.nih.gov/pubmed/23063021
- https://nutritionfacts.org/2015/09/24/exercise-as-medicine/
- https://www.cancer.gov/about-cancer/causes-prevention/risk/obesity/physical-activity-fact-sheet